To Vaccinate or Not to Vaccinate Your Child?

OrangeBooks Publication

1st Floor, Rajhans Arcade, Mall Road, Kohka, Bhilai, Chhattisgarh 490020

Website: **www.orangebooks.in**

© **Copyright, 2024, Author**

All rights reserved. No part of this book may be reproduced, stored in a retrieval system, or transmitted, in any form by any means, electronic, mechanical, magnetic, optical, chemical, manual, photocopying, recording or otherwise, without the prior written consent of its writer.

First Edition, 2024
ISBN: 978-93-5621-624-2

TO VACCINATE OR NOT TO VACCINATE YOUR CHILD?

DR.SANDEEP B

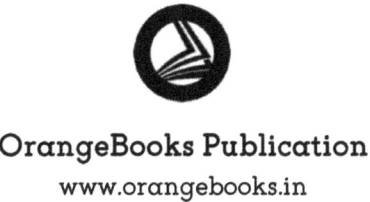

OrangeBooks Publication
www.orangebooks.in

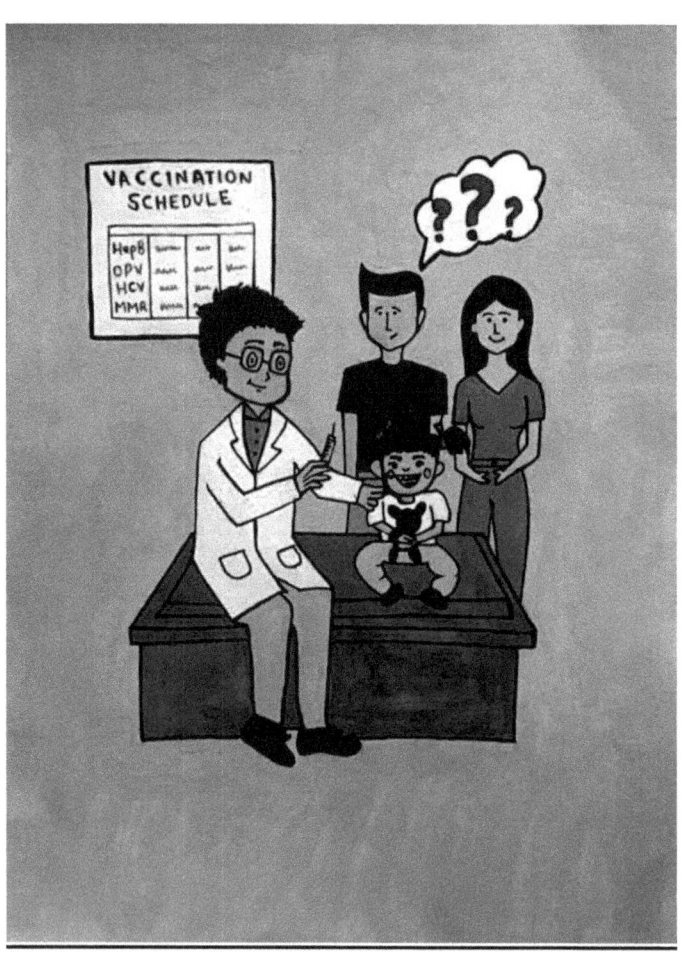

Preface

As a paediatrician, having been in this field for nearly twenty years, I have seen many caregivers and the parents having constantly ignored the importance of vaccinating their children.

Seeing so many diseases and deaths due to various diseases in the community, I used to think a simple prick in the form of a timely vaccine would have saved all this.

On an average, I might have given vaccines to more than 200000 children. Whenever a child has been brought for my consultation, I make sure I impart information to the caregiver or the parent on the importance and the necessity of getting the child vaccinated.

In this post covid stricken era, Vaccinating the child becomes even more important as the overall herd immunity (immunity in the community) has come down.

So as to save the life of children and also to prevent them from suffering from various life-threatening diseases, it's our utmost duty to get them vaccinated.

I dedicate this book to all the parents in the community with bundles of queries on immunization. Hope, this will allay their doubts and fears. (Special thanks to Dr. Kusuma for the illustrations).

Dr. Sandeep B Professor and

Chief Consultant Paediatrician

Table of Contents

Preface v

1. History of Vaccines 1

2. Why The Vaccines Were Introduced 3

3. Global Implication of The Vaccines 5

4. Diseases Prevented by The Vaccines 6

5. Diseases Eliminated by The Vaccines 9

6. Why Is There A Proper Immunization (Vaccination) Schedule In Each Country? 10

7. What Should You Do If You Immigrate To A Different Country? 11

8. What Has To Be Done If You Are Traveling To A Country With The Child For A Short Duration? 12

9. Benefits Of Vaccination 13

10. (A) Growth And Development of Children 16

10. (B) Effectiveness of Vaccination 20

11. How do vaccines act 21

12. Actual Vaccination 22

13. Can Vaccines Cause Any Of The Diseases That They Are Meant To Protect Against? 23

14. What Are Combination Vaccine And Are They Efficacious & Safe?..24

15. Preparation For Vaccination 25

15. (A) One Week Before Vaccination Things To Be Done At Home 26

15. (B) One day prior to the vaccine, things to be done 29

15. (C) On the day of the vaccination.................................30

16. Other Things To Be Done In The OPD..........................33

17. To Be Noted 34

18. Immediately After Vaccination, Things to Be Done .35

19. Can Vaccines Cause Side Effects?...................................36

20. (A) Do Vaccines Hurt? 37

20. (B) Can Vaccines Cause Swelling? 38

20. (C) If So, Why Do The Vaccines Cause Swelling?......39

20. (D) How long will the swelling last post vaccination if it has occurred? 40

20. (E) What Has To Be Done If The Swelling Occurs? 41

20. (F) How To Do Cold Compress? 42

20. (G) How Long The Cold Compress To Be Applied? 43

20. (H) How to prepare a cold compress?.........................44

20.(I) How To Prepare An Ice Pack? 45

20.(J) What to do if pain or swelling or discomfort at the injection site still persists after the compresses? 46

20. (K) When Should You Worry About The Swelling Or Pain? 47

20. (l) Why Not Hot Compresses At The Injection Site? 48

20.(M) Remedies to be used at home for the side effects. 49

20.(N) When To Consult the Doctor For The Side Effects? 50

20.(O) Any Contradictions For The Vaccination 51

21. COVID and VACCINATION 52

21. (A) Covid Positive mother? 53

21. (B) Covid Positive Child? 54

21.(C) Covid Vaccines For Children 55

21.(D) Special Conditions 56

21.(E) Regular Vaccination During Post Covid Times 57

22. What Is The Recommended Schedule Of Vaccination Of Anti-Rabies Vaccines In Children? 58

23. Conclusions 59

24. Bonus Section 60

1.
History Of Vaccines

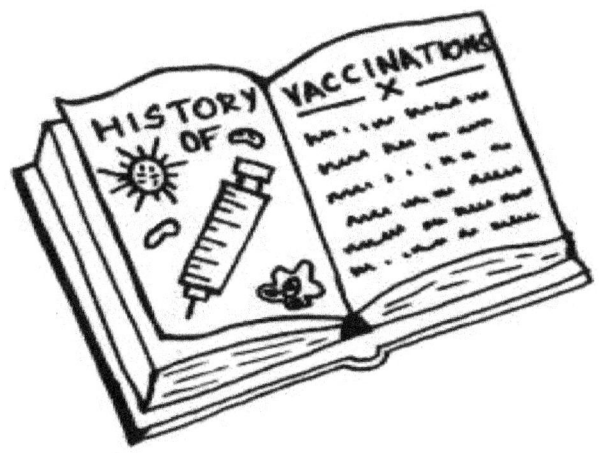

As early as 200 BC, the first vaccine originated in the form of an inoculum (a healed infectious portion of skin or scab from a healed person) introduced into a new person so that, that person would develop immunity before contracting the disease. For instance, this was first employed in the case of small pox.

To Vaccinate Or Not To Vaccinate Your Child?

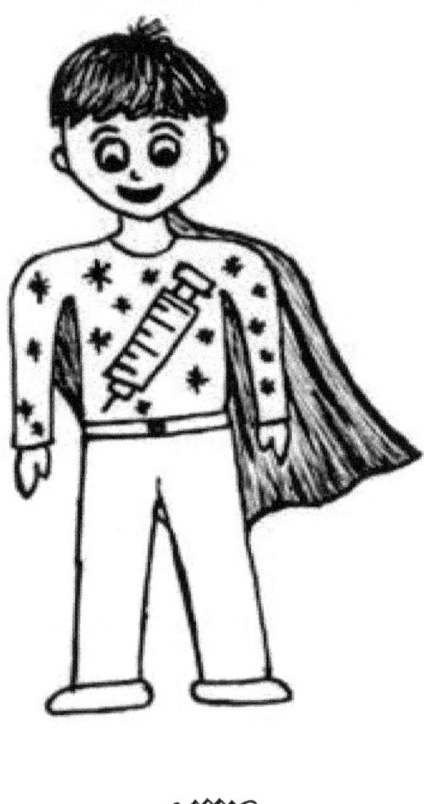

2.
Why The Vaccines Were Introduced

As seen in the history

Following various outbreaks from the fifteenth century till the present date, epidemics like the small pox outbreak, the Spanish pandemic, whooping cough epidemic in Paris, Measles epidemic in Boston, plague in India, each of these had claimed millions of lives. The requirement for something concrete on a large scale was the need of the hour to prevent people from dying in large numbers. Then came the blessings in the form of Edward Jenner, who was the great person who coined and found out the first vaccine (small pox), and following the above trail, other vaccinations for various diseases like polio, chicken pox, rubella emerged consequently.

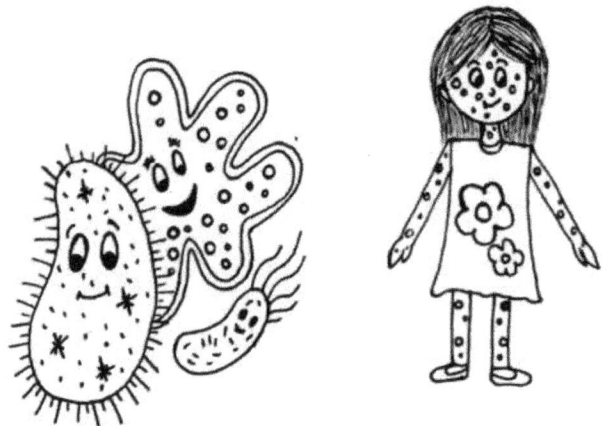

In nineteenth century, in children, there were some diseases which used to lead to deaths in large numbers like Diphtheria, Tetanus, Pertussis, Polio, Measles, Rubella, Haemophilus Influenza type b, Influenza, Rotavirus, Typhoid, Tuberculosis and Pneumococcal infections. The production of vaccines for these diseases brought down the mortality (death rate) drastically.

3.

Global Implication Of The Vaccines

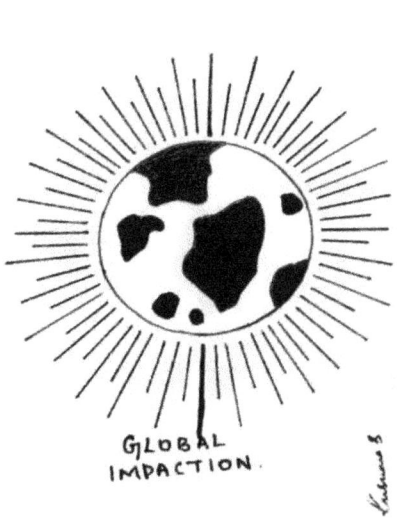

In the last ten years, more than 1 billion children have been vaccinated.

Currently routine immunizations, have been reducing around 3 million deaths every year.

4.
Diseases Prevented By The Vaccines

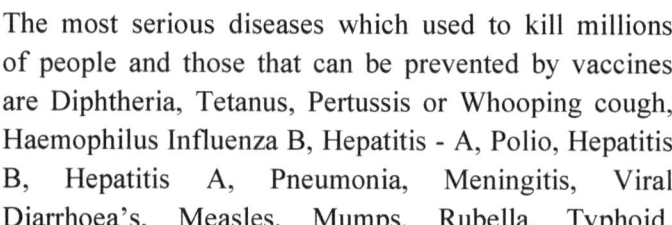

The most serious diseases which used to kill millions of people and those that can be prevented by vaccines are Diphtheria, Tetanus, Pertussis or Whooping cough, Haemophilus Influenza B, Hepatitis - A, Polio, Hepatitis B, Hepatitis A, Pneumonia, Meningitis, Viral Diarrhoea's, Measles, Mumps, Rubella, Typhoid, Yellow Fever.

In developing countries, Tuberculosis which was in endemic proportions was reduced by the BCG vaccine which is indeed given now in majority of these countries.

Certain diseases like Diptheria, Whooping cough and Pertussis which used to cause deaths in large amounts in children and prolonged stay in the hospitals were prevented drastically by the vaccines and were totally eradicated in some countries.

Measles was a viral infection which used to cause fever of high grade with rashes and in certain developing countries, people due to their traditional practices, used to keep the child at home for a week and eventually in certain cases as the severity of the disease used to increase, it used to cause death of the child. This disease was also brought down drastically by the introduction of the Measles vaccine.

An infection called Rubella used to cause deafness, hearing loss and heart defects in children leading on to affect the quality of life in a majority of children and also in some cases used to require surgical corrections of the heart leading on to a huge expenditure and loss of time for the caregivers. Hence, in the first instance, if the child had been immunised with a vaccine which is less than 2 dollars, thousands of dollars to the family could be avoided!

Meningitis – Infection of the brain caused by certain organisms like Streptococcus Pneumonia, N. Meningitidis, H. Influenza, Group B Streptococcus is a serious infection which can cause high degree of fever, convulsions (fits)and if not treated even death of the child or long term complications like inability to walk, speech abnormalities, vision defects. —Just following a routine schedule of vaccines would bring down all these conditions.

Rotavirus is a major virus which is still one of the leading causes of under-five mortality that is death of children less than five years of age, commonly it used to cause loose stools and vomiting in children. Just a simple vaccine has brought down this infection by drastic numbers.

Human Papilloma Virus (HPV) Vaccine given to Pre-Adolescent girls prevents incidence of Cervical Cancer when they grow up, as around 90 % of the cervical cancers are caused by HPV.

In this post Covid stricken era, many queries are being raised about the vaccination against Influenza virus which is very important as this helps to protect the child against the seasonal flu which usually leads on to common cold, cough and later on severe infections. If a child has received two doses of influenza vaccine, within the first year of life, a booster dose that is one dose every year till five years of age is enough to provide sufficient amount of immunity. Every year based on the strain of the influenza virus, the vaccines are produced to offer protection against that particular strain and other common strains which are always prevalent.

Poliomyelitis is a disease in children which causes a crippling condition where the child if gets affected, won't be able to walk for life long. This is prevented by just a few doses of polio vaccine (as per the recommendations, at least five doses by 5 years of age) and in some countries just two drops of the vaccine. In spite of this disease being eradicated in many countries, if the overall vaccine coverage rate drops down, an endemic of this disease can occur, which might be a matter of concern.

5.

Diseases Eliminated by The Vaccines

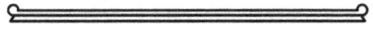

With the advent of vaccines, certain diseases have been eliminated in certain countries, for example in US, six major diseases which once had taken millions of life have been totally eliminated now and they are Small Pox, Polio, Diptheria, Mumps, Measles and Rubella.

6.

Why Is There a Proper Immunization (Vaccination) Schedule in Each Country?

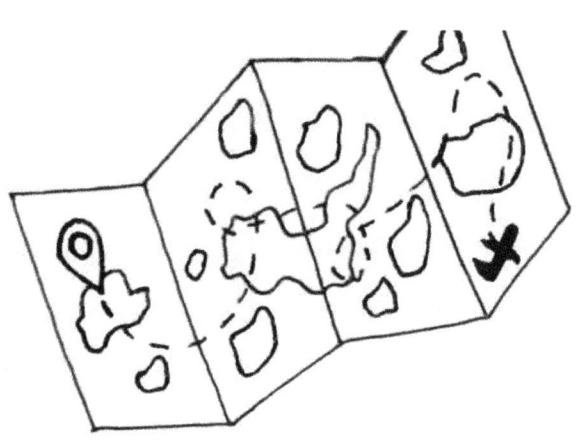

Every country has certain diseases, which are specific to that country apart from common diseases affecting worldwide and also some diseases infect the child more at a particular age, hence after decades of research by health professionals, a proper schedule or timings have been postulated. Therefore, following a stipulated schedule is very important.

7.
What Should You Do If You Emigrate To A Different Country?

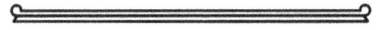

Due to various reasons, if you migrate to a different country with your child, there is nothing to panic. Before leaving the country, kindly contact your regular Paediatrician and take a clear and detailed account or record of your child's vaccination and present it to your concerned Child Specialist at the new country that you have migrated to. Majority of the vaccines are common to many countries, only the schedules or patterns might be different. Kindly enquire about any extra vaccines that the child has to receive as certain diseases might be more prevalent in that region.

8.

What Has To Be Done If You Are Traveling To A Country With The Child For A Short Duration?

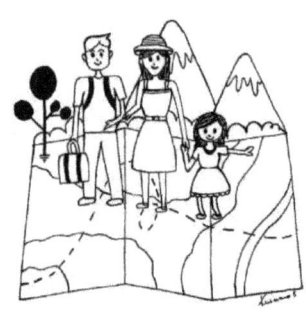

If the child has been immunized as per the schedule of your country, only a few vaccines have to be given before traveling to a new country and this depends on the additional diseases that are prevalent in that Nation, for instance, if a trip is planned to some countries, certain vaccines like MMR (Measles, Mumps, Rubella Vaccine) is mandatory, certain countries also mandate yellow fever vaccine, Polio vaccine, Hepatitis A Vaccine, Malaria Vaccine as a part of the protocol for the travel.

9.
Benefits Of Vaccination

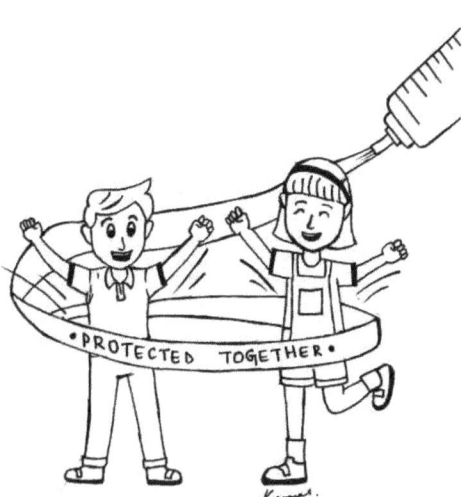

Prevention of Serious diseases

Diarrhoea

Pneumonia

Typhoid

Tetanus

Brain infections (Meningitis, Encephalitis) Severe Viral infections like Measles, Chicken Pox, Flu (Influenza), Hepatitis A, Hepatitis B, Polio, Rubella.

Prevention of Spread of Diseases

When a large number of children get vaccinated in a community, they are healthy, won't get infected, hence won't spread the disease to the unvaccinated children who are vulnerable to get the disease and also, vaccinated children spread the non- infectious strain of the organism, which tends to spread in the environment and protects even the non- vaccinated children against the infectious strains of the organism. (called as Herd Immunity).

Prevention of Epidemics

Each of the diseases which have been listed above have caused a large number of pandemics before and all these have been avoided recently by the vaccines thereby preventing death of millions of children and adults worldwide.

Prevention of Disabilities

Many of the diseases have known to cause a lot of disabilities in children and this has been prevented by the discovery of vaccines against them. To quote a few- Hearing disability, Visual abnormality (Congenital Cataract) and congenital heart diseases used to be caused by Rubella virus and this has been prevented by the advent of the Rubella Vaccine.

Polio Virus used to cause crippling disabilities in children where children used to have weakness of lower limbs and difficulty in walking and this disease has been totally eradicated in most of the countries by a simple Polio Vaccine.

There are some infections of the Brain like meningitis and encephalitis, from which if there is a partial recovery can cause defects in the child, like weakness of limbs or vision disturbances or speech abnormalities and this was largely prevented by vaccines like Hib Vaccine and Pneumococcal vaccines.

Some viral illness like Chicken pox once it heals can leave permanent scars on the skin of the child and such diseases can be prevented in the first place by the vaccine.

10. (A)

Growth And Development of Children

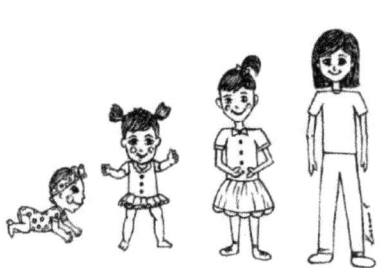

While children keep suffering from diseases on a regular basis, it might hamper their growth and development as during the days of illness, the child might not consume normal regular nutritious food. Certain diseases like Measles have a vicious cycle, like a child with malnutrition or under nutrition is more prone to get measles and a child who has got measles on the long run can go to a state of malnutrition (due to less consumption of food during the illness).

For instance, in developing countries a virus called as rotavirus causes severe loose stools and vomiting and when a child keeps getting affected by it on a regular basis, it will on a long run lead to malnutrition and in turn hamper the growth and development of that child.

Schooling

Vaccinating a child reduces the sick days and absenteeism from school due to common infections like Influenza (Flu), Chicken Pox, Measles.

Communicable diseases (diseases which can spread from one person to the other) like chicken pox, measles, influenza, can cause illness not only in the affected child but also in all the children that this child would have come in contact during the incubation period, which in certain cases, the child might have gone through without any symptoms at all. The child might have attended school normally and have played with the other children while still harboring the infectious agent and spreading the disease to other children. Majority of these communicable diseases are prevented by the vaccines.

Delayed Schooling

Vaccinating a child can indirectly prevent delayed schooling. In some developing countries, diseases like Polio cause crippling illness in children where the child won't be able to walk and in certain brain infections after being treated, the child might have some residual defects or weakness and all these might cause delayed starting of school.

Productivity of children

Vaccination will lead to healthy children and these pupils are always healthy and happy not only at their homes but also at their schools and in their surrounding environment. They would eat well, play well, study well and sleep well. They would grow up to become healthy disease-free adults which in turn is highly productive for a Nation.

Economic benefits at the country level

Vaccination is a great boon for the financial aspect of a country, for example in India, the introduction of Rotavirus vaccine has prevented an estimate of around 20 million dollars for the nation, which used to be spent on the treatment of the same previously.

In the last decade treatment costs for Pneumonia due to the introduction of the vaccine has been reduced by around 1.3 billion US dollars.

It has been found that even if there is a vaccination coverage of around 90 % against some diseases it can save millions of dollars for the country and this money can be used for other developmental projects in the country.

Economic benefits at the caregiver and the family level.

Vaccines prevent a large number of diseases, If a child who has not been vaccinated gets a disease, this will lead on to a burden on the earning parent, who has to spend more money to get the medicines and also for doctors consultation or hospitalization.

Any simple hospitalization for a disease like diarrhea (loose stools) would surmount to a minimum of 100 to 200 dollars expenditure in the simple scenario where as a vaccine costing as less as around 10 dollars on an average would have saved the entire infection by about 90 percent. (resembling the famous quote- a stitch in time saves nine)

On the household...

In majority of the middle-income group families every month there is a pattern set for normal expenditures like food, clothing, shelter and some amount for certain recreations or entertainments. When a child falls sick, if the family have not done insurance for the child or have not planned well, a majority of the money goes in here for which the compensation is either in one of the basic amenities or if there is another sibling that sibling's wellbeing and care getting affected.

Parents have to take off from their work to care for the younger ones and if it's a prolonged illness then they might lose their job also.

10. (B)

Effectiveness of Vaccination

In majority of cases, vaccines offer 90 to 100 percent immunity against serious diseases provided they have been taken on time and as per the schedule and in some cases, even if the vaccine has not been able to prevent the disease per se, it will prevent the major complications of the disease. In case of a viral infection called Measles, Vaccine not only prevents the disease but also its complications like Pneumonia, Meningitis (Brain Infection). BCG vaccine which is given in some countries, might not fully prevent Tuberculosis but it will prevent the various life-threatening complications of Tuberculosis.

In cases, where the vaccine has not given full 100 % protection to the child, still if the child gets exposed to the same infectious agent which the vaccine was supposed to prevent on the first instance, the symptoms will be usually very mild compared to that of a child who has not been immunized at all.

In order to be effective, some vaccines need to be given only once where as others in two or more doses with a fixed interval between them for better immunity and protection.

11.

How Do Vaccines Act

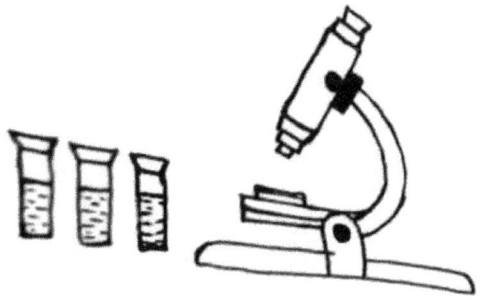

How vaccines work

Basically, our body has defense mechanism against disease causing bacteria and viruses by producing substances called as antibodies.

Vaccines inject inactivated pathogens (infectious agents) like bacteria or viruses (since they are inactivated, they can't produce infection but provoke the production of antibodies). Now if the person gets exposed to real bacteria or viruses and if they enter the body, these antibodies which are already present there will fight against the new bacteria or viruses and would kill them and thus would prevent the infection.

12.

Actual Vaccination

The vaccine or injection in children is usually given to the thigh on the upper aspect by deep intramuscular route. The doctor or the person administering the vaccine sterilizes the area first and then injects the vaccine and following vaccination, applies deep pressure to prevent any minor negligible bleeding that might occur when the needle is withdrawn from the site.

13.

Can Vaccines Cause Any Of The Diseases That They Are Meant To Protect Against?

No, Vaccines never will as such cause any disease that they are meant to protect against.

14.

What Are Combination Vaccine And Are They Efficacious & Safe?

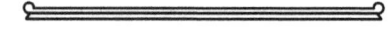

Combination Vaccine means a vaccine which contains a combination of several vaccines combined together and given in a single shot or a single prick.

They are absolutely safe and equally efficacious like the individual vaccines given separately.

The main advantage is that it avoids many pricks for the child and also avoids many visits to the Out Patient Department of the Hospital especially.

15.

Preparation For Vaccination

As in the life of the child, as well as the parent or caregiver, the day of vaccination can be a big day as the child, as well as the caregiver would have several questions and doubts in their minds.

There are certain things which if done prior to the visit to the outpatient department, will decrease the anxiety or apprehension about the vaccine in the minds of the child and the parent and make both of them well prepared for the same.

15. (A)

One Week Before Vaccination Things To Be Done At Home

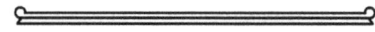

Based on the age of the child

Newborn child

Make sure the child is taking feeds well, avoid any unnecessary travel or getting exposed to any illness from other siblings or from other members at home or at outside.

In case of a bigger child (1 to 5 years)

Make sure the child is on a healthy diet, free from any infections, avoid the contact of this child with any sick child in the neighborhood.

Prepare the child mentally for the vaccine in the following ways –

Enacting

In front of the child, act yourself at one time as the adult or the caregiver.

Other time as the doctor who is injecting the vaccines.

Third time as the nurse who is holding the child.

Role play or Enacting

Play a simple game with the child in the manner the child understands –

Play a pretend game where in you (caregiver) make the child act as the doctor and you enact as the child. Now take a plastic play syringe and ask the child to inject into you and act as if there was a very little pain during the procedure. Then explain to the child that it was totally fine and that you had experienced a very mild pain.

Switching over

Now enact as if you are the doctor and the child as the child itself and gently explain to the child like a doctor would do and make the child lie down and slowly pretend injecting with a plastic syringe into the child. Once this is done, ask the child if he/she felt any pain and explain that it is absolutely fine.

Child (5 to 10 years)

Role models

Children of this age group will be constantly playing with dolls or would have got influenced with some animated characters like Barbie in case of girls and Avengers in case of boys.

Search for any videos where their favorite cartoon characters have gone to some clinics or hospitals and have received vaccine and are looking happy and cheerful after having received the injection. This will motivate the children to a great extent since they would be trying to imitate everything the character does.

Children (Above 10 years)

This age group of children will be more understanding and would need just the explanation as to why they are being injected, the diseases that are prevented by the vaccine and if they dont get the vaccine and acquire the disease, the consequences that they have to undergo in the form of various medications, injectable drugs and the number of days that they won't see or play with their friends or eat food of their choices.

Peer influence

If there is an elder sibling in the house who has received the vaccine, make that sibling to explain to this child that the experience of vaccination is a smooth one and that there will be very minimal pain during the shot or vaccine.

Community — friends

Usually, children above five years will always have their own group of friends. Make other children in the group who have received the vaccine to explain to this child, that it is absolutely fine to receive the injection and that only minimal pain is present during the shot.

15. (B)

One Day Prior To The Vaccine, Things To Be Done

One day before vaccination things to be done to prepare the child mentally for vaccination.

Make sure you give the child a healthy diet preferably home food and as far as possible avoid travel and coming in contact with any sick child or sick adult and ensure that the child has slept well before the day of the vaccination.

15. (C)

On The Day Of The Vaccination

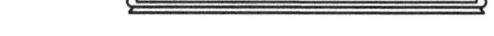

Timings to reach the Opd

At least make sure, you are in the Opd of the doctor half an hour before receiving vaccines so that the child gets accustomed to the hospital surroundings.

Almost every Opd has a baby feeding room, In case of infants less than six months of age, feed them once half an hour before receiving the vaccines.

For children between six months to one year also, reach at least fifteen minutes before your consultation time so that the child slowly gets over the fear of the surroundings.

Same thing applies to children more than one year.

In the OPD/ Hospital

Favoritism

By the time your child reaches an age of six months, you would be able to read the mind of the child in the form of the things that would make them happy in the form of a favorite toy or a short video or a short rhyme or some song which they adore and would feel extremely happy when it's being played or shown.

keep the so-called favorite thing ready and use it as a means of distracting the child as soon as the vaccine is being administered.

Reward technique

In case of infants from birth to six months of age, however, after vaccination, direct breast feeding is the best reward for the child as emotionally it soothes the child.

In bigger children, a chocolate that they usually like or a small new toy of their interest, would keep them happy and won't make a fuss as they will have in their minds that they will be rewarded if they cooperate during the vaccination.

Breathing technique

In case of an older child, like more than five years of age, ask the child to be continuously taking deep breaths during vaccination as this will distract the child totally from the vaccination.

Behaviour –Parent/Caregiver

Parents or accompanying care givers should never show any signs of fear or anxiety in front of the child being vaccinated as children can pick up the instincts very fast and it will in turn enhance their unnecessary fear and doubts and might lead to panic.

Accompanying caregiver or parent should have a calm peaceful attitude during the entire process of the immunisation.

Sib help

If the child has an elder sibling, make that child speak to the one who is about to receive the vaccine in the OPD and motivate this child and explain to the child that, it's going to be easy. This will build a moral boost to the child as in most of the things the younger child tends to follow the elder one.

16.

Other Things To Be Done In The OPD

As soon as you enter the Opd or examination room with your child, first greet or wish the doctor. Seeing this your child will be more comfortable and at ease with the doctor.

17.

To Be Noted

If you have something to be told about the child or if you have basic doubts regarding diet or growth aspects or some other doubts about the past illness of the child it's better you ask them before the vaccine is done so that once the vaccine is given, the child might become uncooperative or start crying and it becomes extremely difficult both for the doctor and the caregiver to calm the child or focus on other details.

18.

Immediately After Vaccination, Things to Be Done

The doctor would have kept the swab at the injection site. Hold the swab with a minimal gentle pressure for at least thirty seconds. In case of a new born, after

five mins of vaccination, feed the child, which in turn acts as the best analgesic (pain killer). In case of a bigger child try to keep telling the child that everything is ok, now there is no pain, ask the child to be taking deep breathes which acts as a diversion technique and would in turn pacify the pain.

19.

Can Vaccines Cause Side Effects?

Common side effects of vaccines are mild pain, redness and swelling at the site of vaccination. Usually, it's self-limiting and subsides within a few hours and rarely needs any medical intervention.

In about 99 percent of the cases, vaccines don't have any side effects at all. Only in rare cases a few side effects are noted at the site of injections, like mild pain and in some cases mild swelling.

Both these features last only for a few hours and is self-resolving.

In certain countries, where still some diseases like Tuberculosis are rampant, there is a vaccine called as BCG vaccine, which is usually given to the left hand and after its administration, it gives rise to a small swelling and later a small wound like lesion and finally a permanent small mark or a scar, this is the normal course and the parents or the care givers should not show any apprehension towards it.

20. (A)

Do Vaccines Hurt?

Yes, vaccines do hurt very little just in the form of just a pin prick for a mild moment.

How long does the pain from a vaccine remain?

In majority of the vaccines, the pain will persist for less than ten seconds.

In which type of vaccine, the pain might persist longer?

Only in some vaccines like DPT, the pain might persist a little longer but usually subsides within half an hour. With the advent of newer type of this vaccine called DTap, the pain is negligible hence, it's also called as the painless vaccine.

20. (B)

Can Vaccines Cause Swelling?

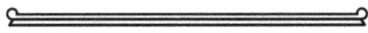

No

In very rare cases, say one in ten thousand children, some vaccines might cause a mild swelling.

20. (C)

If So, Why Do The Vaccines Cause Swelling?

In Ninety nine percent of the cases it's due to the faulty technique of administering the vaccine.

20. (D)

How Long Will The Swelling Last Post Vaccination If It Has Occurred?

Maximum only for a day or two.

20. (E)

What Has To Be Done If The Swelling Occurs?

Cold fomentation or cold compresses over the site is the best thing to be done.

20. (F)

How To Do Cold Compress?

A neat cold wet cloth can be applied at the injection site which is painful or has swollen or an ice pack can also be applied as an alternative. An ice pack or a cold compress will reduce the pain and the swelling at the site.

20. (G)

How Long The Cold Compress To Be Applied?

Ideally speaking for a total duration of two to three mins per sitting.

Most importunately, continuous compressions should not be given. It has to be given intermittently, for instance, compression has to be given for ten seconds, a gap of ten seconds has to be given and again it has to be continued.

20. (H)
How To Prepare A Cold Compress?

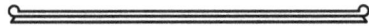

Wet a neat clean cloth with pure clean water and put this cloth in a neat sterile polythene bag and place this bag in the freezer for a duration of five mins and then remove it for usage.

20.(I)
How To Prepare An Ice Pack?

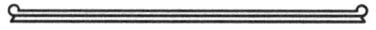

Take a neat sterile towel, put ice cubes taken from the refrigerator into that towel and wrap it around and now it's ready to be used. This cloth can be put inside a sterile polythene bag.

20.(J)

What to do if pain or swelling or discomfort at the injection site still persists after the compresses?

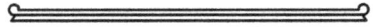

Use a mild topical analgesic (cream or ointment applied at the injection site) after consulting your doctor or a mild oral analgesic in the form or drops or syrup or tablet in consultation with your doctor.

20. (K)

When Should You Worry About The Swelling Or Pain?

If the swelling persists or becomes thickened and remains so even after three days after vaccination you have to consult your doctor or if the child continues to cry due to pain or uneasiness from the vaccine even after an hour of receiving the vaccine, you have to consult the doctor.

20. (I)

Why Not Hot Compresses At The Injection Site?

Ideally heat will cause vasodilatation, that is, it will increase the blood supply at the site, so it is ideal to give hot compression before vaccination for better absorption of the vaccine.

Usually, hot compresses can be used in aches or spasms in children following sports injuries as this will help in eliminating the various toxic metabolic products in the muscle which would have accumulated during exercise or the sports activity.

20.(M)

Remedies to be used at home for the side effects

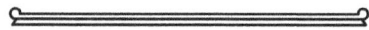

As mentioned above, cold compresses and in rare cases analgesic local application at the site of injection.

20.(N)

When To Consult the Doctor For The Side Effects?

If the side effects like pain, swelling or redness are severe or are causing severe discomfort to the child in the form of excessive inconsolable crying even after feeding and comforting or if the pain or swelling has lasted for more than two days then immediately a paediatrician has to be consulted.

20.(O)

Any Contradictions For The Vaccination

Are there any contradictions for the vaccination?

In the new born period, jaundice is not at all a contradiction for the routine vaccination

In children common cold, cough are not at all a contradiction.

Only in case of high-grade fever or severe loose stools, vaccination is at the discretion of the paediatrician. Some immunocompromised states like cancer, HIV or in children on certain medications like steroids are cases of relative contradictions and vaccination is done after discussion with the Paediatrician.

21.
COVID and VACCINATION

21. (A)

Covid Positive Mother?

If the mother of the new born is Covid positive and if the child is not symptomatic and Covid test report is negative then the child can be immunized with routinely scheduled vaccines.

21. (B)

Covid Positive Child?

Once the child recovers from the illness and has been tested negative and is totally asymptomatic, the child can undergo routine immunization.

21.(C)
Covid Vaccines For Children

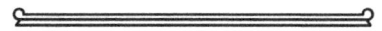

Recent recommendations

All children, five years of age and above have to receive one dose of an updated COVID-19 vaccine.

Children between 5 to 11 years who are not vaccinated or have received one dose of COVID-19 vaccine before September12, 2023 have to receive one updated COVID-19 vaccine.

Children of age 12 and above who are not vaccinated before should receive either one or two doses of COVID-19 vaccine based on the brand and as per recommendations.

(Source-CDC)

21.(D)

Special Conditions

If a child was without symptoms and was in the incubation period for the covid infection and has unknowingly received the vaccine even then it's safe as the routine vaccine given to this child won't affect the disease process.

21.(E)
Regular Vaccination During Post Covid Times

Routine vaccinations during post covid times should never be withheld, as during the covid era, many of the routine vaccines had not been received by the children due to lockdown or covid illness, henceforth, bringing down the overall immunity of the children and making them susceptible to the diseases.

Certain diseases are always are on the verge of out breaks like influenza and measles and vaccination prevents these diseases to a large extent. If the immunization coverage for these illnesses have dropped down, then the children are at a greater risk of acquiring them.

22.

What Is The Recommended Schedule Of Vaccination Of Anti-Rabies Vaccines In Children?

Since children love pets like cats and dogs a lot, hence there is a tendency of them being bitten or scratched by them accidently while playing with them. The standard schedule is five doses on days 0, 3, 7, 14 and 30, with day '0' being the day of commencement of vaccination. The first dose should be administered as soon as possible after exposure. Usually in children, based on the type of vaccine either 0.5 ml or 1 ml intramuscularly can be given.

23.
Conclusions

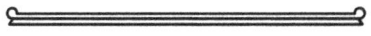

As we approach the end of this book, we have realised the importance of getting the child vaccinated. So as a parent or a caregiver if we really adore our child it's our duty and responsibility to get our child vaccinated.

24.
Bonus Section

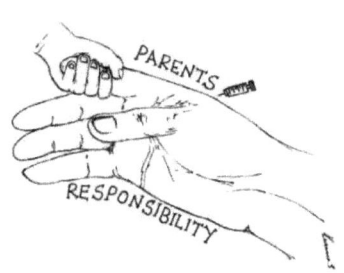

Questions to be asked to the Paediatrician before the vaccine is given-

1. Which vaccine will be given on that particular day.
2. Cost of the vaccine.
3. About the schedule or the date for the next visit for the vaccine.
4. Any side effects of the vaccine like pain or swelling.
5. If any side effect occurs, after how much time after the administration of the vaccine those side effects might occur.

6. What precautions have to be taken to avoid the side effects.

7. What are the things to be done once the side effects occurs.

8. Any medications that the doctor would prescribe anticipating the side effects.

9. How much time after receiving the vaccine, the child should be in the Opd for any observation.

10. When can the child be fed after immunization — in case of an infant — when the child can be direct breast fed and in case of a toddler or preschool or school age child how much time later, the child can be given solid or liquid diet.

11. If any side effects after the vaccine occur, whom to contact in the hospital premises later.

12. Contact number of some resourceful person in the hospital.

13. Always maintain and carry the vaccine record of the child.

14. If you are visiting a regular Paediatrician, kindly send the picture of your immunization card showing previously given vaccines and the current vaccine which has to be given as it will help the doctor to procure the vaccine if it's not available at present.

www.ingramcontent.com/pod-product-compliance
Lightning Source LLC
LaVergne TN
LVHW061621070526
838199LV00078B/7376